Rajiv Mathur

Pediatric And Neonatal Drug Doses

Rajiv Mathur

Pediatric And Neonatal Drug Doses

LAP LAMBERT Academic Publishing

Impressum / Imprint

Bibliografische Information der Deutschen Nationalbibliothek: Die Deutsche Nationalbibliothek verzeichnet diese Publikation in der Deutschen Nationalbibliografie; detaillierte bibliografische Daten sind im Internet über http://dnb.d-nb.de abrufbar.

Alle in diesem Buch genannten Marken und Produktnamen unterliegen warenzeichen-, marken- oder patentrechtlichem Schutz bzw. sind Warenzeichen oder eingetragene Warenzeichen der jeweiligen Inhaber. Die Wiedergabe von Marken, Produktnamen, Gebrauchsnamen, Handelsnamen, Warenbezeichnungen u.s.w. in diesem Werk berechtigt auch ohne besondere Kennzeichnung nicht zu der Annahme, dass solche Namen im Sinne der Warenzeichen- und Markenschutzgesetzgebung als frei zu betrachten wären und daher von jedermann benutzt werden dürften.

Bibliographic information published by the Deutsche Nationalbibliothek: The Deutsche Nationalbibliothek lists this publication in the Deutsche Nationalbibliografie; detailed bibliographic data are available in the Internet at http://dnb.d-nb.de.

Any brand names and product names mentioned in this book are subject to trademark, brand or patent protection and are trademarks or registered trademarks of their respective holders. The use of brand names, product names, common names, trade names, product descriptions etc. even without a particular marking in this work is in no way to be construed to mean that such names may be regarded as unrestricted in respect of trademark and brand protection legislation and could thus be used by anyone.

Coverbild / Cover image: www.ingimage.com

Verlag / Publisher:
LAP LAMBERT Academic Publishing
ist ein Imprint der / is a trademark of
ICS Morebooks! Marketing SRL
4, Industriala street, 3100 Balti, Republic of Moldova
Email: info@omniscriptum.com

Herstellung: siehe letzte Seite /
Printed at: see last page
ISBN: 978-3-330-33391-8

PEDIATRIC & NEONATAL

DRUG DOSES

DR R C MATHUR

Consultant Pediatrician

Hyderabad

Dedicated to

My father Prof Y C Mathur, a doyen & my inspiration

My great mother Madhur Mohini

My wife Swati, my backbone

My gems Ria & Jai

INDEX

ACETAMINOPHEN (PARACETAMOL)

Neonates – oral /rectal 10-15mg/kg/dose 6-8hourly as needed. Max: 40mg/kg/day

Infants & children – oral 10-15 mg/kg/dose 4-6hourly as needed

Rectal 1-20 mg/kg/dose 4-6 hourly as needed

Children >12 years – oral 10-15 mg /kg/dose 4-6hourly as needed

Rectal 10-20 mg /kg/dose 4-6 hourly as needed

Toxic dose: > 4gm/day

Toxic blood concentration for hepatotoxicity: > 200 mcg/ml at 4 hours post ingestion

> 50 mcg/ml at 12 hours post ingestion

ACETYLCYSTEINE (N- ACETYLCYSTEINE)

Acetaminophen (Paracetamol poisoning): Begin treatment within 8 hours of ingestion when the serum concentration is above the "Possible" level on the Modified Rumack Mathew Normogram given below.

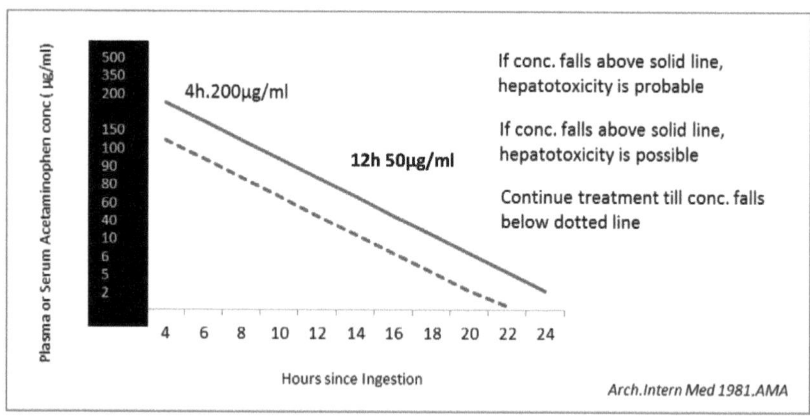

Treatment should also be started in children when there is an acute ingestion of > 150mg/kg in a child & > 7.5gm in an adolescent.

First dose : 150mg/kg in 200ml 5% dextrose over 1 hour , Second dose: 50mg/ kg in 500ml 5% dextrose over 4 hours, Third dose : 100mg/kg in 1000ml 5% dextrose over 16 hours.

Nebulized inhalation:

Infants: 1-2 ml 20% solution or 2-4 ml of 10% solution, 6-8 hourly

Children: 3-5ml 20% solution or 6-10 ml 10% solution 6-8 hourly

Adolescents: 5-10ml of 10-20% solution 6-8 hourly.

Children should receive nebulized bronchodilator 15 minutes before acetylcysteine.

ACYCLOVIR

Genital herpes simplex virus: Oral: 40-80mg /kg/day 4 divided doses for 5-10 days.max 1g/day

IV: 5mg/kg/dose 8 hourly for 5-7 days

HSV in immunocompromised host: oral 1g/day in 4 divided doses for 7-14 days max 1g/day

IV: < 12yrs 10mg/kg/dose 8hourly for 7-14 days,

IV: > 12 yrs 5mg/kg/dose 8 hourly for 7-14 days

HSV encephalitis: children 3months to 12 yrs: 20mg/kg/dose 8 hourly for 14-21 days

>12 yrs 10mg/kg/dose 8 hourly 14-21 days

Neonatal HSV: IV 20mg/kg/dose 8 hourly 14-21 days

Varicella in immunocompetant host: Oral: 20mg/kg/dose for 5 days.

(Initiate within 24 hours of onset of rash)

Varicella zoster in immunocompromised host: 10mgkg/dose 8 hourly 7-10 days or until 48hrs of

Zoster in immunocompetant host: oral 20mg/kg/dose 4 times a day for 7-10 days.

ADAPALENE

Acne: children > 12 Yrs: Topical 0.1% gel, everyday night to avoid photosensitivity.

ADENOSINE

Neonates, Children <50kg: 0.05-0.1 mg IV. If not effective than incremental dose every 2 minutes by 0.05mj/kg or until termination of SVT. (max6mg)

ALBENDAZOLE

INDICATION	DOSE	DURATION
Neurocysticercosis	15mg/kg/day, 2 divided doses (max 800mg/day)	8-10 days
Hydatid disease	15mg/kg/day, 2 divided doses	28 days
Ascariasis, Anchylostoma	400mg stat	single dose
Cutaneous larva migrans	400 mg single dose	3 days
Trichonella spiralis	400mg twice daily	8-14 DAYS
Visceral larva migrans	400mg twice a day	3 days
Enterobious vermicularis	400mg single dose, repeat after 2 weeks if needed.	

ALBUMIN

5% Albumin for hypervolemia

20% Albumin for hypoproteinemia

0.5-1g/kg/dose infused over 3-4 hours. May repeat every 1-2 days.

ALBUTEROL (SALBUTAMOL)

Nebulization:

Acute severe asthma: wt< 20kg 0.5ml in 3ml NS   > 20kg 1mlin 3ml NS every 20 minutes for 3 doses, then every 1-4 hours as needed. Continuous nebulized salbutamol 0.3mg/kg/hour in life threatening acute severe asthma.

Less severe asthma: 0.15mg/kg/dose 1-4 hourly.

MDI with spacer

Less severe asthma 4 puffs every 20 minutes for 3 doses, then every 1-4 hourly.

Maintenance:

 1-4 years 1-2 puffs every 4-6 hours as needed

>5years 2 puffs every 4-6 hours as needed.

Exercise induced bronchospasm: 1-2 puffs 5 minutes before exercise.

Oral salbutamol: 1month-2years 0.3-0.4 mg/kg/day

2-6 years: 1mg every 8 hourly

6-12years: 2mg every 8 hourly

>12 years 2-4mg every 8 hourly

AMBROXOL

1.2-1.6mg/kg/day ((30mg/5ml liquid formulation)

1-2 years: 2.5ml BID

3-6 years: 5ml TID

7-12 years: 2to 3 times a day

>12years 5ml TID

AMIKACIN

Neonates; 0-4 weeks: <1200 gm – 7.5mg/kg/dose every 18-24 hourly

1200-2000 gm- 7.5mgkgdose 12 hourly

>2000 gm – 7.5-10mg/kg/dose 12 hourly

Infants & children: 15-20mg/kg/day divided into 8 hourly doses.

AMOXICILLIN

Oral

Neonates & infants ≤ 3months: 20-30mg /kg/day in divided doses 8hourly

Infants ≥ 3 months & children: 25-50mg /kg/day in divided 8 hourly doses or 12 hourly doses

Acute Otitis Media: 80-90mg /day in divided 12 hourly doses

Community acquired pneumonia: 80-100mg /kg/day in divided 6-8 hourly doses

Endocarditis prophylaxis: 50mg/kg dose 1 hour before procedure.

AMOXICILLIN AND CLAVULANIC ACID

Oral: (based on Amoxicillin component)

 Neonates & infants ≤ 3 months: 30 mg/kg/day in divided 12 hourly doses

 Children: 25-45 mg/kg/day in divided 12 hourly doses

I.V: (based on Amoxicillin component)

 Children 0-3 months: ≤ 4kg: 30mg /kg /day in divided 12 hourly doses

                    ≥ 4kg: 30mg/kg/day in divided 8 hourly doses

Children 3 months to 12 years: 30 mg/kg /day in divided 6-8 hourly doses

Children ≥ 40kg: 1.2 gm in divided doses 6-8 hourly

AMPHOTERICIN B LIPOSOME

Infants ≥ 1 month & children:

Empiric therapy: 3mg/kg/day once daily infusion over 2 hours

Systemic fungal infection: 3-5 mg /kg/day once daily infusion over 2 hours

Cryptococcal meningitis in immune compromised: 6mg/kg/day once daily infusion over 2 hours

AMPICILLIN

Oral; Children: 5-100mg/kg/day in divided doses 6 hourly (max 3gms/day)

IV; Neonates ≤ 7 days: 50-75 mg/kg/day in divided doses 12 hourly

    Meningitis: 100-150 mg/kg/day in divided doses 8-12 hourly

   Neonates > 7 day: 50-100mg/kg/day in divided doses 6,8 or 12 hourly

    Meningitis: 100-200mg/kg/day in divided doses 6-8 hourly

Group B Streptococcal meningitis: 300mg/kg/day in divided doses 6 hourly

Infants & children: IM or IV: 100-200mg/kg/day in divided doses every 6 hourly

Meningitis: 200-400mg/kg/day in divided doses every 6 hourly

Endocarditis prophylaxis: 50mg/kg dose 30 minutes before dental, oral, respiratory tract or esophageal procedure

For Genitourinary procedure add Gentamycin 1.5mg/kg dose

AMPICILLIN AND SULBACTUM

I.M/I.V:

Infants ≥ 1 month: 100-150mg/kg/day of Ampicillin in divided doses 6 hourly

Meningitis: 200-300mg/kg/day in divided doses every 6 hourly

Meningitis: 200-400mg/kg/day in divided doses 6 hourly (max 8gms)

ANTIHEMOPHILIC FACTOR (RECOMBINANT- rAHF)

The dose has to be individualized based on the coagulation profile

1IU/kg of rAHF raises factor VIII by 2%.

Formula to calculate dose based on the desired increase in factor VIII (% of normal)

IU required = body wt. (kg) × 0.5×desired increase in factor VIII (IU/dl or % of normal)

General dosing:

Minor hemorrhage: (required AHF level: 20-40%) 10-20IU/kg every 12-24 hourly, for 1-3days

Moderate hemorrhage: (required AHF level: 30-60%) 15-30IU/kg every 12-24 hours for 3-4 days

Severe life threatening hemorrhage: (required AHF level 80-100%) 40-50IU /kg first dose then 20-50 IU/kg every 8-12 hourly until bleeding has resolved

Minor surgery: (required AHF level 30-80-%) 15-40 IU /kg dose 1 hour prior to surgery. Repeat dose if needed 8-24 hourly

Major surgery: (required AHF level 80-120%) 40-60I/kg 1 hour before procedure. Repeat dose if needed 8-24 hourly

ANTI RETROVIRAL DRUGS FOR HIV

Class of drug	Antiretroviral drug	Dose
NRTI	Abacavir (ABC)	16mg/kg in 2 divided doses
NRTI	Didanosine(ddl)	240mg/m2 in 2 divided doses
NRTI	Emtricitabine(FTC)	6mg/kg once a day
NRTI	Lamivudine(3TC)	8mg/kg in2 divided doses
NRTI	Stavudine (d4T)	2mg/kg in 2 divided doses
NRTI	Tenofovir(TDF)	8mg/kg once a day
NRTI	Zidovudine (AZT/ZDV)	8mg/kg in 2 divided doses
NNRTI	Efavirenz (EFV)	15mg/kg once a day
NNRTI	Nevirapine(NVP)	2weeks:120mg/m2 once a day then 240-400mg/m2 in 2 divided doses
PI	Lopinavir/Ritonavir(LPV/r)	450mg lpv+115rtv/m2 in 2 divided doses
PI	Nelfinavir((NFV)	110-130mg/kg in 2 divided doses
PI	Ritonavir(RTV)	Initial:400mg/m2 slowly increase to 800mg/m2 in 2 divided doses
FUSION INHIBITOR	Enfuvirtide	SubQ >6years:4mg/kg in 2 divided doses

NRTI: Nucleoside reverse transcriptase inhibitors NNRTI: Non Nucleoside reverse transcriptase inhibitors PI: Protease inhibitors

ARTEMETHER AND LUMEFANTRINE

Oral: To be taken after food

Children 2months to <16 years

5-≤ 15 kg: 0 hour 1 tablet/2.5ml, after 8 hours1 tablet/2.5ml & day 2 &3 1 tablet/2.5ml BID for 2 days

15-≤ 25kg: 0 hour 2 tablet/5ml, after 8 hours 2 tablets/5ml & day 2 &3 2 tablets/5ml BID for 2 days

25-≤ 35 kg : 0 hour 3 tablet /7.5ml, after 8 hours 3 tablets/7.5ml & day 2 &3 3 tablets BID/7.5ml for 2 days

≥ 35 kg: 0 hour4 tablet/10ml, after 8 hours 4 tablets/10ml & day 2 &3 4 tablets/10,l BID for 2 days

ARTESUNATE

IV or IM

Loading dose; children ≤20 kg 3mg/kg, ≥ 20kg 2.4mg/kg

Then after 4 hours; 1mg/kg, 24 hours; 1mg/kg

 Day 3 onwards: 1mg/kg once a day oral/IV/IM for maximum 7 days.

Reconstituted in 5% sodium bicarbonate & diluted in equal volume of Normal saline or

5% dextrose.

Oral

Children ≥ 6months: 5mg/kg day 1, 2.5mg/kg on day2 &3 as single daily dose. On day 2 combine with Mefloquin 15mg/kg dose

ASCORBIC ACID (VITAMIN C)

Recommended adequate intake 0-6 months: 40 mg, 6-12 months: 50mg

Recommended daily allowance:

1-3 years: 15mg, 4-8 years: 25mg, 9-13 years: 45mg, 14-18 years 70mg

Scurvy: 100-300mg in 2 divided doses

Dietary supplementation: 35-50 mg/day

ASPIRIN

Analgesic; oral: 10-15 mg /kg/dose every 4-6 hours max 4gms/day

Anti-inflammatory; oral initial: 60-90mg/kg/day in 3 divided doses, maintenance 80-100mg/kg in 3- 4 divided doses

Antiplatelet effects: oral: 3-5mg/kg/day single daily dose.

Kawasaki Disease; Oral: 80-100mg/kg/day in 4 divided doses up to 14 days, then 3-5mg/kg/day once daily for > 7 weeks.

ATENOLOL

Oral:0.8mg-1mg/kg/day max 100mg/day

ATOMOXETINE

Children ≥ 6years: 0.5mg /kg/day increase to max 1.2mg/kg/day or max 100mg/day, whichever is lower, after 3 days

ATORVASTATIN

Hyperlipidemia & hypercholesterolemia: > 10 years; 10mg once a day

ATROPINE

Organophosphate or Carbamate poisoning

IV 0.02-0.05 mg/kg every 10-20 minutes until Atropine effect(dry flushed skin ,tachycardia, fever, mydriasis) is seen ,then every 2- 4 hours for at least 24 hours

Bradycardia

IV or Intratracheal: 0.02mgkg. Minimum dose 0.1mg, maximum dose 0.5mg in children & 1mg in adolescents. May be repeated every 5 minutes.

AZATHIOPRINE

Inflammatory bowel disease (Crohns disease); Oral: 3mg/kg/dose once daily

Transplantation; oral/IV: initial 3-5mg/kg/day single daily dose, maintenance 1-3mg/kg/day single daily dose

Lupus Nephritis; oral: 2-3mg/kg/once daily dose

Rheumatoid arthritis: oral; 1mg/kg/once daily dose for 6-8 weeks, if needed increase 0.5mg/kg every 4 weeks max 2.5mg/kg/day. Minimum 12 weeks of treatment for adequate response trial.

Monitor WBC count weekly, Renal & liver function tests bi weekly.

AZELASTINE

Seasonal allergic rhinitis: 1 spray in each nostril twice a day

Vasomotor rhinitis > 12 years: 2 spays twice a day

AZITHROMYCIN

Infants; oral: 10mg/kg/once single daily dose. 5 day course for Pertussis

Children > 6months:

Respiratory tract infection: 10mg/kg/once daily dose 3-5 days

Community acquired pneumonia: 10mg /kg once daily dose for 5 days or 30mg /kg single dose

Otitis media: 10mg /kg once daily dose for 5 days or 30mg /kg single dose

Pertussis: 10mg /kg once daily dose for 5 days

Acute bacterial sinusitis: 10mg /kg once daily dose for 3-5 day

Children ≥ 2 years

Pharyngitis, Tonsillitis: 10mg/kg/once daily dose (max 500mg) for 5 days

Prevention of bacterial endocarditis: 15mg/kg single dose 1 hour prior to procedure

Chancroid: single 20mg /kg dose. Max 1gm

Uncomplicated chlamydial urethritis: single 20mg/kg dose Max 1gm

Prevention of chronic pseudomonas infection: 250mg on Monday, Wednesday, Friday.

Adolescents

Bacterial sinusitis: 500mg once daily for 3 days

Community acquired pneumonia, Pharyngitis, Tonsillitis, skin infections, exacerbation of COPD: 500mg/once daily for 5 days

Chlamydia trachomatis urethritis, cervicitis: 1 gm. single dose

Endocarditis prophylaxis: 500mg single dose 1 hour prior to the procedure

AZTREONAM

IM or IV

Neonates

≤ 7days; ≤ 2kg 60mg/kg/day in 2 divided doses, ≥ 2kg 80mg/kg/day in 3 divided doses

≥ 7 days; <1.2kg 60mg/kg/day in 2 divided doses ,1.2-2kg 90mg/kg/day in 3 divided doses, > 2kg 120mg/kg/day 6 hourly divided doses

Children > 1 month: 90-120mg/kg/day in 3-4 divided doses (max 8gms/day)

BECLOMETHASONE

Dose should be selected based on the severity of disease & patient response. Start with the lowest dose.

IM; Children: Adrenocortical deficiency (physiological replacement):0.0175-0.125mg base/kg/day in 2-4 divided doses.

Adolescents: 0.6-9mg/day as a single or 2divided doses.

Oral; Children: Adrenocortical deficiency (physiological replacement): 0.0175-0.25mg/kg/day in 3-4 divided doses.

Adolescents: 2.4-4.8mg/day in 2-4 divided doses.

BIOTIN

RDA: 100-200mcg/day.

Biotin deficiency: 5-10mg once a day.

BISACODYL

Oral: Administer on an empty stomach

Children3-12 years: 5-10mg or 0.3mg/kg as single dose.

Children > 12years: 5-15mg/day single dose

Rectal suppository: Children < 2 years: 5mg as single dose

Children 2-11 years: 5-10mg as single dose

Children > 12 years: 10mg as single dose

BUDESONIDE

Intranasal: Children > 6 years: 2 sprays once a day. Max: 4 sprays /day

Oral Inhaler with spacer: 200-400 mcg puffs twice a day

Nebulization: 0.25mg-0.5mg 12th hourly

Oral for mild to moderate Crohns disease: 0.45mg/kg single dose. Max: 9mg/day. Dissolve nebulizer solution in 15ml water.

BUDESONIDE & FORMOTEROL

Maintenance treatment for Asthma:

Children: 2 puffs 12th hourly

CAFFEINE

Apnea of prematurity: oral /IV:

Loading: 10-15mg/kg as caffeine citrate (5-10mg/kg as caffeine base).

 Maintenance dose: caffeine citrate 5mg/kg/day (2.5mg/kg /day as caffeine base) once a day 24 hours after loading dose.

CALCITRIOL

Hypocalcaemia in CKD: oral

  < 10kg: 0.05mcg alternate days

 10-20kg: 0.1-0.15mcg daily

 >20kg: 0.25mcg daily

Hypoparathyroidism/pseudohypoparathyroidism: oral

 <1year: 0.04-0.08mcg/kg daily once

 1-5 years: 0.25-0.75mcg once daily

 >6years:0.5-2mcg once daily

Vitamin D Dependent Rickets: oral 1mcg once daily

Vitamin D Resistant Rickets: initial dose: 0.015-0.02mcg once daily,

                        Maintenance: 0.03-0.06mcg/kg once daily max 2mcg.

Hypocalcaemia of prematurity: oral: 1 mcg/day for first 5 days of life

Hypocalcemic Tetany of prematurity: IV 0.05mcg/kg once a day for 5days

CALCIUM SALTS

Oral CALCIUM SALT	ELEMENTAL CALCIUM mg/g salt	CALCIUM meq/g salt
Calcium acetate	250	12.7
Calcium carbonate	400	20
Calcium chloride	270	13.5
Calcium citrate	211	10.6
Calcium glubionate	64	3.2
Calcium gluconate	90	4.5
Calcium lactate	130	6.5
Calcium phosphate tribasic	390	19.3

RDA < 6months: 400mg/day

6-12 months: 600mg/day

1-10years:800mg/day

11-24 years: 1200mg/day

Hypocalcaemia; oral. Dose as elemental calcium (Max 1gm)

  Neonates: 50-150mg/kg/day in 4-6 divided doses

  Children: 45-65mg/kg/day in 4 divided doses

Calcium gluconate IV:

Tetany: 100-200mg/kg/dose over 5-10minutes as an infusion. Dose may be repeated after 6 hours (max 3gm)

Maintenance: Neonates: 3-4mEq/kg/day, Infants & Children: 1mEq/kg/day

Hypocalcemia: IV 200mg/kg/day in 4 divided doses.

Cardiac arrest in Hypocalcemia, hypokalemia, magnesium toxicity: 100mg/kg/dose, can repeat after 10 minutes (max3gms)

CARBAMEZAPINE

15-20mg/kg/day (max 35mg/kg/day. 12-15years 1gm/day, >15 years1.2gm/day). In 2-3 divided doses

CARNITINE

Oral: 50-100mg/kg/day in 2-3 divided doses (max 3gms/day)

CEFACLOR

Children > 1month: 20-40mg/kg/day every 2-3 divided doses (max 2gm/day)

Lower dose for Pharyngitis & a higher dose for Otitis media.

CEFADROXIL

30mg/kg/day in 2 divided doses. (Max 2g/day)

CEFAZOLIN

IM or IV

Neonates: <7days: 40mg/kg/day in 2 divided doses. > 7days 40-60mg/kg/day in 3 divided doses

Infants & children: 25-100mg/kg/day divided every 6-8 hourly.max 6g/day

Bacterial endocarditis prophylaxis in penicillin allergic: for dental & upper respiratory procedures: 1g 30minutes before procedure.

CEFDINIR

Oral

>6months to 12 year: 14mg/kg/day in 2 divided doses. 5-10days

> 12 years: 300mg BID for 5-10days.

CEFEPIME

IM, IV

Neonates < 14 days: 30mg/kg/dose 12th hourly.   > 14 days: 50mg/kg/dose 8th hourly

Children: 50mg/kg/dose every 12th hourly

Febrile neutropenic patients: 50mg/kg/dose every 8th hourly

CEFIXIME

Oral

Infants & children: 8mg/kg/day divided every 12 hourly (max 400mg/day)

Treatment of acute UTI: 16mg/kg/day divided 12hourly doses on day1, then 8mg/kg/day single daily dose for 13 days.

CEFOTAXIME

IV/IM

Neonates 0-4 weeks: 100-150mg/kg/day in 2 divided doses

Infants & children till 12years: 100-200mg/kg/day in 2-3 divided doses

Meningitis: 200mg/kg/day in 4 divided doses

CEFOXITIN

IV

Neonates: 100m/kg/day in 3 divided doses

Infants: 100-160mg/kg/day in 3 divided doses (max 12g/day)

CEFPODOXIME

Oral

Infants & children <12years: 10mg/kg/day in 2 divided doses (max 800/day)

>12years: 100-400mgdose every 12 hourly

CEFPROZIL

Oral

Infants & children up to 12 years: (max 1g/day)

Pharyngitis & tonsillitis; 15mg/kg/day in 2 divided doses

Otitis media: 30mg/kg/day in 2 divided dose

>12 years: 250-500mg every 12 hourly

CEFTAZIDIME

IM/IV

Neonates: 0-4 weeks: 100mg/kg/day divided every 12 hourly

Infants & children up to 12 years: 100-150mg/kg/day every 8 hours (max6g/day)

Meningitis: 150mg/kg/day in 8hourly divided doses

CEFTIZOXIME

IV

Infants >6months &children: 150-200mg/kg/day divided 6-8 hours. (max 12g/day)

CEFTRIAXONE

IV/IM

Neonates: 50mg/kg/day as single daily dose.

Infants & children; 50-75mg/kg/day divided every 12-24hours

Acute bacterial Otitis media: 50mg/kg as single dose, if persistent for 3 days

Meningitis: 100mg/kg/day every 12-24 hours.max 4g/day for 14 days

Epiglotitis: 50-100mg/kg once daily for 2-14 days

Typhoid fever: 100mg/kg/day every 12-24 hours for 5-14 days

Lyme disease: 75-100mg/kg/day for 2-4 weeks

Uncomplicated Gonoccocal infection: 125mg as single dose

Chancroid: 50mg/kg as single dose

Acute Epidydimitis: 250mg as single dose

CEFUROXIME

IV

Neonates: 50-100mg/kg/day divided 12 hourly doses

Children: 75-150mg/kg/day divided 8 hourly doses. Max 6g/day.

CEFUROXIME AXETIL

Oral

Infants >3months – children up to 12 years: 20-30mg/kg/day max500mg/day in 2divided doses

Children >12years: 250mg 12 hourly

CEPHALEXIN

Oral

Children: 25-50mg/kg/day divided 6-8 hourly

Severe infections, Otitis Media, uncomplicated cystitis 50-100mg/kg/day divided 6-8hourly

Endocarditis prophylaxis: 50mg/kg single dose 30minutes before procedure.

CETRIZINE

Oral

Children 6-12 months: 2.5mg once a day

Children 1-2 years: 2.5mg every 12 hours

Children 3-5years:2.5-5mg every 12 hours

Children > 6years: 5-10mg every 12 hours

CHARCOAL ACTIVATED

Oral

In water/sorbitol

Infants (only in water): 1g/kg

Children: 1-12 years: 1-2g/kg (25-30g). 1g adsorbs 100-1000g of poison

Children >12years:30-100g

Only Activated charcoal in water can be used in multiple doses every 2- 6 hourly till clinical symptoms of poison decrease or ileus develops.

CHLORAL HYDRATE

(Triclofos 500mg/5ml)

Oral: sedation: 30-60minutes prior to non painful procedures (EEG, CT Scan/MRI)

Neonate: 25mg/kg/dose

Infants & Children: 25-50mg/kg/dose. Max dose infants 1g, children 2g

CHLORAMPHENICOL

50-100mg/kg/day in 3-4 divided doses. Max 4g/day

For Enteric Fever give for 14 days & for meningitis for 3 weeks.

CHLOROQUIN

Oral after food

Prophylaxis for Malaria: 5mg/kg base /as one dose a week .start 1-2 weeks prior to travel & 4 weeks after travel.

Treatment of Malaria: 0 hour: 10mg/kg/dose. After 6 hours,24 hours,48 hours:5mg/kg/dose

CHLORPHENIRAMINE MALEATE

Children <12 years: 0.35mg/kg/day in divided 4-6 hourly doses

(2-5 years: 1mg every 4-6 hours; 6-12 years: 2mg every 4-6 hours. max 12mg/day)

Children > 12 years: 4mg every 4-6 hours.max 24mg/day

CHOLESTYRAMINE

240mg/kg/day in 3 divided doses with meals.max 8g/day

CHORIONIC GONADOTROPIN

IM

Prepubertal cryptorchidism

4000units 3times a week for 3 weeks/ 5000units every second day for 4 injections/500units 3 times a week for 4-6 weeks

Hypogonadtrophic hypogonadism

500-1000units 3 times a week for 3weeks then same dose twice weekly for 3 weeks/1000-2000units 3 times/ week , 4000units 3 times /week for 6-9 months, reduce to 2000units/week for another 3 months.

CIPROFLOXACIN

Neonates: IV: 7-40mg/kg/day in 2 divided doses, in susceptible septicemia

Children: Oral: 20-30mg/kg/day in divided 12 hourly doses max 1.5g/day

IV: 20-30mg/kg/day in divided 12 hourly doses max 1g/day

UTI, Pylonephritis: 10-21 days, Bone & joint infection: 4-6 weeks, Cystic fibrosis: 4-6 weeks, infectious diarrhea: 5-7 days, Typhoid fever: 10-14 days, Inhalation Anthrax: 60 days, LRTI: 7-14 days.

Ophthalmic: 1-2 drops every 2-6 hourly

CITRATE AND CITRIC ACID

Oral; 2-3mEq/kg/day or 5-15ml diluted in water 6-8 hourly, after meals.

CLARITHROMYCIN

Oral

15mg/kg/day in 12 hour divided doses

CLEMASTINE

Oral

Infants & children <6 years: 0.25-0.5mgbase/kg/day in 2-3 divided doses.max 1mg base/day

Children 6-12 years: 0.5-1mgbase/kg/day.max 3mg base/day

Children > 12 years;1-2mg base 3 times a day.max 6 mg base/day

CLINDAMYCIN

IV

Neonates <7days: 10-15mg/kg/day divided every 8-12 hourly

Neonates> 7days:10-30mg/kg/day divided every 6-8 hourly

Infants & children: 25-40mg/kg/day divided every 6-8hourly. Oral: 10-30mg/kg/day divided 6-8hourly.max1.8g/day

Adolescents: IV: 1.2-2.7g/day in 2-4 divided doses. Oral: 15-450mgdose every 6-8 hours.

CLONAZEPAM

Oral

Infants & children<10years or 30kg

 Initial:0.01-0.03mg/kg/day in 2-3 divided doses can increase by 0.5 mg every other day.max 0.05mg/kg

 Maintenance dose: 0.1-0.2mg/kg/day in 3 divided doses. Max 0.2mg/kg/day

Children >10 years or >30 kg

 Initial: 1.5mg in 3 divided doses

 Maintenance dose: 0.05-0.2mg/kg/day max 20mg/day

CODEINE

Oral

Analgesic: 0.5-1mgkg/dose every 6hourly max 60mg/dose

Antitussive :> 2years: 1-1.5mg/kg/day in 6 hourly divided doses

Or 2-5 years: 2.5-5mg (max 30mg/day)every 6 hourly, 6-12 years:5-10mg(max 60mg/day) every 6 hourly,>12years: 10-20mg/dose (max 120mg/day)every 6 hours

CYANOCOBALAMIN

RDA: 0-6months: 0.4mcg/day, 7-12months:0.5mcg/day, 1-3 years: 0.9mcg/day, 4-8years: 1.2mcg/day, 9-13 years: 1.8mcg/day, >14years: 2.6mcg/day.

Pernicious anemia:

Neonates & infants: IM.0.2mcg/kg for 2 days, 1000mcg/day for 2-7 days the maintenance 100mcg/month

Children; IM: 30-50mcg/kg (total 1000mcg/day), maintenance: 100mcg/day

CYCLOPHOSPHOMIDE

Non hematological problems:

Oral: 2-8mg/kg/day in 2 divided doses

IV: 10-15mg/kg in 2 divided doses

CYPROHEPTADINE

Oral

Allergy: 2-6 years: 2mg every 8-12 hourly (max12mg/day), 7 to 14 years: 4mg every 8-12hourly (max 16mg/day).

Cluster headaches & migraine: 4mg 2-3 times a day

CMV IMMUNE GLOBULIN

Prophylaxis for Renal & liver transplant: IV: 150mg/kg within 72hrs before transplant 100mg/kg at weeks 2,4,6,8, then 50mg/kg at week 12, 16.

Prophylaxis in Bone Marrow Transplant: IV 200/kg given 6& 8 days prior to transplant & on day1, 2, 8 then 200mg/kg on days 14, 21

DEFEROXAMINE

Acute iron intoxication: serum Iron levels >500mcg/dl .IV:15mg/kg/hour.max 12g/day

Chronic iron intoxication: SubQ: 20-50mg/kg/day over 8-12 hours.max 2g/day

DESLORATIDINE

Children 6-11months:1mg once a day

1-5 years: 1.25mg once a day

Children 6-11years: 2.5mg once a day

Children >12 years: 5mg once a day

DESMOPRESSIN

Nocturnal enuresis

Children > 6years: Oral: 0.2mg at bed time. Fluid restriction 1hour before & 8 hours after dose

Diabetes Insipidus: Oral: 0.05mg 2 times a day

DEXAMETHASONE

Neonates

Airway edema/extubation: IV 0.25mg/kg dose 4 hours prior & the every 8 hours 3doses

BPD extubation facilitation: IV 0.5-0.6mg/kg/day in divided 12 hourly doses for 3-7 days

Children

Airway edema/extubation: IV, IM/oral: 0.5-2 mg/kg/day in divided 6 hourly doses, begin 24hours prior & continue for 4-6 doses

Anti-inflammatory: Oral/IM/IV: 0.08-0.3mg/kg/day in divided doses 6-12 hours

Bacterial Meningitis: > 2months age: IV 0.6mg/kg/day divided every 6 hourly .start with antibiotic & continue for 4 days

Cerebral edema: Oral/IM/IV: loading dose:1-2mg/kg dose. Maintenance: 1-1.5mg/kg/day max 16mg/day divided every 6 hourly

DEXTROMETHORPHAN

1-3months: 0.5-1mg every 6-8 hours

3-6months: 1-2 mg every 6-8 hours

7months -2 year: 2-4 mg every 6-8 hours

2-6 years: 2.5-7.5 mg every 6-8 hours

7-12 years: 5-10 mg every 6-8 hours

>12 years: 10-30mg mg every 6-8 hours

DEXTROSE

Hypoglycemia

Neonates: 1-2ml/kg dose of 10% solution followed by continuous infusion at 4-6mg/kg/minute

Infants <6months: 2.5-5ml/kg dose of 10% solution .max 25g/dose

Infants > 6months & children: 5-10ml/kg of 10% solution.max 25g/dose

DIAZEPAM

Status Epilepticus; IV

> 1month–children: 0.1-0.3mg/kg/dose given over 3-5 minutes.max 10mg dose. Can be repeated after 10minutes.

Moderate Sedation: Oral:0.2-0.3mg/kg max 10mg/dose; Adolescents: Oral 10mg/dose

> 45-60 minutes prior to procedure

> Slow IV: 0.05-0.1mg/kg dose over 3-5 minutes; Adolescents: 5mg

Muscle relaxation & anxiolytic: Oral

> Children <5 years: 1-2mg dose every 6 hourly,

> Children >5 years: 5mg dose every 6 hourly

DICLOFENAC

Oral

Children: 2-3mg/kg/day divided 2-3 times a day

DICLOXACILLIN

Oral

25-50mg/kg/day in 6 hourly divided doses.max 2g/day

DICYCLOMINE

Oral

Infants >6months: 5mg/dose 3-4 times a day

Children>1year: 10mg/dose 3-4 times a day

DIGOXIN

Give half of the total digitalizing dose as the initial dose, 2 quarter doses after 6 & 12 hours. Monitor ECG for toxicity changes after 6 & 12 hours. For maintenance dose: children <10 years 12hour divided dose,>10 years single daily dose. IV dose should be infused over 5-10minutes.

Monitor serum Potassium, Magnesium & calcium.

AGE	TOTAL DIGITALIZING DOSE mcg/kg		DAILY MAINTAINANCE DOSE mcg/kg	
	P.O	IV /IM	P.O	IV/IM
Neonates Preterm Term	20-30 25-35	15-25 20-30	5-7.5 6-10	4-6 5-8
1month-2yrs	35-60	30-50	10-15	7.5-12
2-5 years	30-40	25-35	7.5-10	7.5-12
5-10 years	20-35	15-30	5-10	4-8
> 10years	10-15	8-12	2.5-5	2-3

DIPHENHYDRAMINE

Oral

Treatment of phenothiazine dystonic reactions: 5mg/kg/day in divided 6 hourly doses

Moderate to severe allergic reactions: 5mg/kg/day in divided 6 hourly doses

Minor allergic reactions, minor allergic rhinitis, motion sickness & Antitussive:

  Children 2-6 years- 6.25mg every 6 hours

  Children 6-12 years-12.5-25mg every 6 hours

  Children >12 years- 25-30mg every 6 hours

DOBUTAMINE

Stimulates $\beta 1$ receptor: increased contractility & heart rate

IV continuous infusion

Neonates: 2-15mcg/kg/minute   Children: 2.5mcg/kg/minute   max 40mcg/kg/min

Central line(mg/kg to be added in 50ml NS)	Peripheral line(mg/kg to be added in 50ml NS)
15mg/kg,1ml/hour=5mcg/kg/min	15mg/kg,1ml/hour=5mcg/kg/min

DOMPERIDONE

Oral: 0.3mg/kg/dose 2-4 times a day half an hour before feed

DOPAMINE

Stimulates both adrenergic & dopaminergic receptors.

Low dose 1-5mcg/kg/min: dopaminergic; renal & mesenteric vasodilatation.

Intermediate dose 5-15mcg/kg/min: β1adrenergic & dopaminergic stimulation; increased heart rate, cardiac index & increased renal blood flow

High dose >15mcg/kg/min: α adrenergic stimulation: vasoconstriction, increased blood pressure

Central line(mg/kg to be added in 50ml NS)	Peripheral line(mg/kg to be added in 50ml NS)
15mg/kg,1ml/hour=5mcg/kg/min	3mg/kg,1ml/hour=1mcg/kg/min

DOXYCYCLINE

Oral/IV

Children : >8 years: 2-4mg/kg/day divided into 12-24 hour doses. Max 200mg/day

Lyme disease, Q fever, and Tularemia in children >45kg: Oral 100mg every 12 hours, 14-21 days

Chlamydial infections in children > 45 kg: Oral 100mg every 12 hours,7 days

Brucellosis: Oral 2-4mg/kg/day in 2 divided doses 6weeks in combination with rifampin

Rickettsial disease: >45kg: Oral: 100mg every 12 hours for 7-14 days

Anthrax: Initial IV: 5mg/kg/day in 2 divided doses for 60 days in conjunction with 2nd drug

Change to oral when appropriate

ENALAPRIL

0.1mg/kg/day in 1-2 divided doses .max dose 5 mgs

EPINEPHRINE (ADRENALINE)

Stimulates α, β1 & β2 adrenergic receptors causing relaxation of bronchial tree, peripheral vasodilatation & cardiac stimulation. Large doses cause vasoconstriction of vascular & skeletal smooth muscles & pupilary dilation.

Neonate: IV, Intratracheal: 0.01-0.03mg/kg(0.1-0.3ml/kg of 1:10000 solution) every 3-5 minutes Flush with 5ml NS & 5 manual ventilations.

Infants & children:

Hypersensitivity reactions: IM/IV 0.01mg/kg/0.01ml/kg of 1:10000 solution.max 0.5mg. Can be used every 20 minutes or as 0.1mcg/kg/minute infusion in severe reactions. SubQ 0.01ml/kg of 1:1000 solution .max0.5mg

Bradycardia or Asystole: IV O.1ml/kg of 1:10000 solution.max 10ml.May repeat after 3-5 minutes. Intratracheal 0.1ml/kg of 1:1000 solution & flush with 5ml NS & 5 manual ventilations. Max 0.2mk/kg. Maybe repeated after 3-5 minutes.

Inotropic support: Continuous IV infusion 0.1-1mcg/kg/minute

Central line(mg/kg to be added in 50ml NS)	Peripheral line(mg/kg to be added in 50ml NS)
0.3mg/kg , 1ml/hr= 0.1µg/kg/minute	0.1mg/kg 3ml/hr= 0.1µg/kg/min

Nebulization: 0.25-0.5ml of 2.25% racemic epinephrine solution diluted in 3ml NS

ERYTHROMYCIN

Neonates: <1week: 20mg/kg/day in divided doses every 12 hours

>1week: 30-40mg/kg/day in divided doses every 6-8 hours

Infants & Children: 30-50mg/kg/day in divided doses every6-8 hours. Max 2g/day. For Pertussis & Chlamydial infections treat for 14 days.

ESOMEPRAZOLE

Oral

Children 1-11 years: 1mg/kg/once a day, 1 hour before meal for 8 weeks for GERD or NERD

Children> 12 years: 20-40mg once a day, 1 hour before meal for 8 weeks for GERD or NERD

ETHAMBUTOL

15-25mg/kg/once a day with or without food

ETHOSUXIMIDE

15-40mg/kg/day in divided doses every 12 hour

FERRIC GLUCONATE

IV: Children> 6years; serum Ferritin <500ng/ml: 1.5mg/kg in 50ml NS & infused over 1 hour

FERROUS FUMARATE, FERROUS GLUCONATE, FERROUS SULPHATE, IRON POLYMALTOSE COMPLEX, FERROUS ASCORBATE, FERROUS BISGLYCINATE, CARBONYL IRON, HEME IRON

Oral

Prophylaxis 60-100mg elemental iron/day

Mild to Moderate iron deficiency anemia: 3mg elemental iron /kg/day in 1-2 divided doses

Severe Iron deficiency anemia: 4-6mg elemental iron/kg/day in 3 divided doses.

IRON SALT	ELEMENTAL IRON CONTENT % OF SALT FORM
Ferrous fumarate	33
Ferrous gluconate	11.6
Ferrous sulphate	30
Ferrous bisglycinate	25
Ferrous ascorbate	15
Carbonyl Iron	25
Iron Polymaltose complex	15
Heme Iron	11

RDA for Iron:

<5months-5mg

5month-10 years-10mg

11-18 years; Male -12mg, Female-15mg

FEXOFENADINE

Children 6months-<2 years- 15mg twice a day

Children 2-11 years-30mg twice a day

Children>12 years- 60mg twice a day

FILGRASTIM (GRANULOCYTE COLONY STIMULATING FACTOR)

When Absolute neutrophil count (ANC) -<1000/cumm

IV/SubQ

Neonates- 5-10mcg/kg/once a day for 3-5 days in severe sepsis

Children: 5-10 mcg/kg/once a day for up to 14 days/ till ANC>10,000cu mm

FLUCONAZOLE

Oral/IV

Premature neonates <14days: 6mg/kg/day every 72 hours,   > 14 days: every 48 hours

Neonates <14 days: 6mg/kg/day every 48 hours,

Neonates> 14 days & children: 6mg/kg/once a day

FLUNARIZINE

Prophylaxis of migraine:

Oral

3-12 years: 5mg   >12 years: 10mg once a day

FLUTICASONE

Intra Nasal

Children > 4 years: one spray into each nostril(50mcg each nostril) .max 2 spray in each nostril

Oral Inhalation: with Spacer device

Children< 12 years; Low dose: 44mcg/puff 2-4 puffs a day

Medium dose: 44mcg/puff 4-8 puffs a day

High dose: 110mcg/puff > 3puffs a day

Children >12 years; Low dose: 44mcg/puff 2-6 puffs/day

Medium dose: 110mcg/puff 2-4 puffs/day

High dose: 110mcg/puff >4 puffs a day

Topical for > 3 months of age

FLUTICASONE & SALMETEROL

Children 4-11 years: one puff twice a day with spacer device

Children >12 years: 2 puffs twice a day with spacer device

FOLIC ACID

Folic acid deficiency: Oral

Infants: 0.1 mg/day

Children <4 years: upto0.3mg/day

Children>4 years: 0.4mg/day

RDA

Premature infants: 50mcg/day

Neonates up to 6months: 25-35mcg/day

Children 1-3 years: 150mcg/day

4-8 years: 200mcg/day

9-13 years: 300mcg/day

>14 years: 400mcg/day

FORMOTEROL

Children > 5 years: 1 puff twice a day with spacer device

FOSPHENYTOIN

Status Epilepticus

Loading dose: 15-20mgPE/kg   rate: 2mgPE/kg/min

Non Emergent Load: 15-20mgPE/kg   rate: 1mgPE/kg/min

Maintenance dose: 2-4mgPE/kg every 12 hourly   rate: 1-2mgPE/kg/min

FUROSEMIDE

Neonates: IV/IM 1-2mgmg/kg/dose every 12 -24 hours

Infants & children: oral: 2mg/kg every 12 -24hours .max 4 mg/kg

                    IV 1-2mg/kg/dose every6-12 hours

GANCICLOVIR

Slow IV infusion over 1 hour

Congenital CMV infection: Neonates & infants: 12mg/kg/day in divided 12 hourly doses for 6 weeks

GI & liver infections, Retinitis, Pneumonia: Induction: 10mg/kg/day in divided 12 hourly doses for 14-21 days.   Maintenance: 5mg/kg/day as single dose for 7days/week

Prevention of CMV infection in transplant patients: Induction: 10mg/kg/day in divided 12 hourly doses for 1-2 weeks. Maintenance: 5mg/kg/day as single dose for 7days/week

GENTAMICIN

Neonates: IV/IM   Premature<1.2kg:2.5-3.5mg/kg/dose once in 24 hours

                >7days:2.5mg/kg/dose every 8 hourly

Infants & children<5 years: IV/IM 2.5mg/kg/dose every 8 hourly or 5-7.5mg/kg/as single daily dose

Children> 5years:2-2.5mg/kg/dose every 8 hourly or 5-7.5mg/kg/as single daily dose

GLUCAGON

Hypoglycemia, insulin shock therapy: IV/IM

< 20kg: 0.02-0.03 mg/kg   >20kg: 1mg

GLYCERIN

Constipation: Rectal suppository: as single dose

Neonate: 0.5ml/kg/dose

Children < 6 years: 1 infant suppository or 2-5ml of rectal solution as enema

Children >6 years: 1 adult suppository or 5-15ml of rectal solution as enema.

GRANISETRON

IV/oral

Children > 2years: 10mcg/kg/day, 1 hour before chemotherapy

GRESEOFULVIN

Children>2years: 10-20mg/kg/day single or 2 divided doses after meal (fatty meal)

HEPARIN

Line flushing: 10u/ml 2-5ml/flush

TPN: Neonates: 0.5u/ml added to TPN solution

Infants & children: 1u/ml added to TPN solution

Arterial line: 0.5-2u/ml

Peripheral arterial catheters in situ: continuous IV infusion of heparin at concentration 5 units/ml at 1ml /hour

Umbilical artery catheter: Low dose heparin, continuous infusion in concentration 0.25-1u/ml

Systemic heparinization:

Neonates & infants<1 year: Loading: IV infusion 75u/kg over 10 minutes. Maintenance dose: 28u/kg/hour to keep APTT of 60-85 seconds

>1year: Loading: IV infusion 75u/kg over 10 minutes. Maintenance dose: 20u/kg/hour to keep APTT of 60-85 seconds

HUMAN GROWTH HORMONE

Individualized treatment should be done. Treatment to end when expected height is achieved, Epiphysis is fused or the patient seizes to respond. Expected growth should be >5cm/year. Dose increment should be done after 6 months of treatment if growth rate is <2.5cm/year.

SubQ Norditropin: 0.024-0.034(0.07-0.1u)/kg/dose 6 times a week

HYDROCORTISONE

Acute Adrenal Insufficiency:

Infants: IV 1-2 mg/kg bolus then 25-150mg/day as 6-8 hour divided doses

Children: IV 1-2 mg/kg bolus then 150-250mg/day as 6-8 hour divided doses

Anti inflammatory /Immunosuppressive: Infants & children: IM/IV 1-5mg/kg/day as 12 hourly divided doses

Congenital Adrenal Hyperplasia: Oral: Infants 2.5-5mg three times a day, children: 5-10 mg 3 times a day

Glucose refractory Neonatal Hypoglycemia: IV 1-2mg/kg/dose every 6 hours

Shock: Initial: IV 50mg/Kg bolus followed by 50mg/kg infusion over 24 hour

Status Asthmaticus: 5mg/kg bolus. Maintenance 2mg/kg/dose every 6 hourly

HYDROXYCHLOROQUIN

Immune modifier: JRA/SLE/Pemphigus: Oral 3-5mg/kg/day in 1-2 divided doses

HYDROXYZINE

Pruritus: oral : <6 years- 50mg/day in 3 divided doses

>6years- 50-100mg/day in 3 divided doses

Or

2mg/kg/day in 6-8 hour divided doses

IMIPENEM & CILASTATIN

IV dose based on Imipenem component

Neonates; premature & low birth weight: 20-40mg/kg/day every 12 hour divided doses

Term & AGA: 50-75mg/kg/day in divided 8 hourly doses

Infants up to 3months: 100mg/kg/day divided into 6 hour doses

Infants>3months & children: 60-100mg/kg/day divided into 6 hour doses

IMMUNE GLOBULIN. IV

ITP: 400-1000mg/kg/day for 2-5 days (total dose 2g/kg)

CLL: 400mg/kg/dose every 3-4 weeks

Pediatric HIV with hypogamaglobulinemia: 400mg/kg/dose every 3-4 weeks

Gullian Barre syndrome: 400mg/kg/dose daily for 5 days or 1g/kg/day for 2 days

Kawasaki disease: 2g/kg as single dose .If signs & symptoms persist a 2nd dose to be given. Aspirin should be given along with Immune globulin.

Refractory Polymyositis, Dermatomyositis: 2g/kg/month given over 2 days

Chronic inflammatory demyelinating polyneuropathy: 1g/kg/day for 2 days once each month

INDOMETHACIN

For PDA: IV First dose: 0.2mg/kg followed by 2 doses depending on the post natal age

Post natal age of 1st dose< 48 hours: 0.1mg/kg at 12-24 hours interval

Post natal age of 1st dose: 2-7days: 0.2mg/kg at 12-24 hours interval

Post natal age of 1st dose :> 7 days: 0.25mg/kg at 12-24 hours interval

INFLIXIMAB

Crohns disease: 5mg/kg/dose at week 0 & 2

Uncontrolled JRA: 3mg/kg/dose at week 0, 2, 6

INSULIN REGULAR

Onset of action: 30minutes, max effect: 1-5 hours**,**

Type I diabetes mellitus

Initial dose:SubQ:0.2-0.4u/kg/day in divided doses

Maintenance therapy: use intermediate or long acting form of insulin.

Insulin regular can be used as an intensive therapy on daily therapy.

Diabetic Ketoacidosis:

IV continuous infusion: 0.05-0.1u/kg/hour till serum glucose is 80-100mg/dl & acidosis clears.

Then change to SubQ insulin doses.

Hyperkalemia (after treatment with calcium & sodium bicarbonate)

Dextrose 0.5-1g/kg as 25% solution with regular insulin 1 unit for every 5g dextrose ; infuse over 2 hours.

IPRATROPIUM

Inhalation

Neonates: 25mcg/kg/dose 3 times a day

Infants: 125-250mcg 3 times a day

Children: 250-500mcg 3-4 times a day

Maintenance: MDI 1-2 inhalations every 6-8 hours

Nasal spray: 2sprays in each nostril 2-4 times a day

ISONIAZID

Oral: morning single dose on empty stomach (half an hour before food)

Treatment of Tuberculosis: 10 15mg/kg/day

Max dose 300mg/day

ISOTRETINOIN

Oral

Acne: 0.5-2mg/kg/day at bedtime for 15-20weeks or 75%of cysts have decreased.

IVERMECTIN

Oral

Children>15kg

Scabies: 200mcg/kg as single dose

Strongloidiasis: 200mg/kg once daily for 2 days

Onchochocerciasis: 150mcg/kg as a single dose

Cutaneous larva migrans: 200mcg/kg once a day for 2 days

Pediculosis: 200mcg/kg as single dose.

Trichuriasis: 200mcg/kg once daily for 3 days

Weight based dosage to provide 150mcg/kg	
Patient weight in kg	Single oral dose in mg
15-25	3
26-44	6
45-64	9

Weight based dosage to provide 200mcg/kg	
Patients weight In Kg	Single oral dose In mg
15-24	3
25-35	6
36-50	9
51-65	12

KETAMINE

Slow IV (rate: 0.5mg/kg/minute; minimum time for infusion 1minute)

0.5-2mg/kg/dose

As continuous infusion: sedation: 5-20mcg/kg/minute .Titrate the dose in an incremental method.

KETACONAZOLE

Oral: 3.3-6.6mg/kg/single daily dose

Shampoo: 1minute application twice a week .Minimum 3 days gap between applications

Topical: apply 1-2 times a day

KETOROLAC

2-16 years for analgesia

 Oral: 1mg/kg as single dose

 IM: 1mg/kg max 30mg single dose

 IV: 0.5mg/kg max: 15mg as single dose

>16 years

 Single dose treatment: IM 60mg, IV 30mg

 Multiple dose treatment: IM/IV 30mg 6hourly.max 120mg/day

 Oral 10mg 6 hourly .max 40mg/day

Ophthalmic: seasonal allergic conjunctivitis: 1drop 4 times a day

LACTOBACILLUS SPECIES

5 Billion CFU 2-4 times a day

LACTITOL

Daily single dose

Constipation: 2-6 years: 10ml   >6 years: 10-15ml

Prevention of hepatic encephalopathy: 30ml daily single dose/45-90ml in 3 divided doses till 2-3 loose stools appear

LACTULOSE

Constipation: <1year: 5ml, 1-5 years-10ml, 5-12 years- 20ml, >12 years: 30ml as single or two divided doses

Hepatic encephalopathy: 30-50ml /dose 3 times a day till 2-3 loose stools appear

LAMIVUDINE

Oral

HIV

 Neonates: <30 days: 2mg/kg/dose twice a day

 Infants1-3 months: 4mg/kg/dose twice a day

 Infants>3months-children < 16 years: 4mg/kg/dose twice a day .max 150mg/12hours

 HIV post exposure prophylaxis: in combination with other retroviral or protease inhibitor based on risk 15Omg/dose twice a day

Chronic Hepatitis B: 2-17 years: 3mg/kg/day single dose max 100mg/day

LAMOTRIGINE

As add on therapy: Oral

Use dose adjusted to the immediate lower tablet dosage form, as a whole tablet.

Children 2-12 years

 Add on to Valproic Acid

 Week 1& 2:0.15mg/kg/day in 2 divided doses,

 Week 3&4:0.3mg/kg/day in 2 divided doses

 Maintenance: 1-3mg/kg/day in 1-2 divided doses(max 200mg/day). To achieve this, Increment should be 0.3mg/kg/day every 1-2 weeks added to the earlier daily dose

Add onto phenytoin/carbamezapine

 Week 1&2:0.6mg/kg/day in 2 divided doses

 Week 3&4:1.2mg/kg/day in 2 divided doses

Maintenance: 5-15mg/kg/day in 2 divided doses (max 400mg/day). To achieve this, Increment should be 1.2mg/kg/day every 1-2 weeks added to the earlier daily dose

Add on to Non enzyme inducing & non Valproic acid

Week 1&2:0.3mg/kg/day in2 divided doses

Week 3&4:0.6mg/kg/day in 2 divided doses

Maintenance dose: 4.7.5mg/kg/day in 2 divided doses (max300mg/day). To achieve this, Increment should be 0.6mg/kg/day every 1-2 weeks added to the earlier daily dose

Children>12 years

Add on to Valproic Acid

Week 1& 2:25mg alternate days

Week 3&4:25mg/day

Maintenance: 100-200mg/day in 1-2 divided doses. To achieve this, Increment should be 25-50mg/day every 1-2 weeks added to the earlier daily dose

Add onto phenytoin/carbamezapine

Week 1&2:50mg/day single dose

Week 3&4:100mg/day in 2 divided doses

Maintenance: 300-500mg/day in 2 divided doses. To achieve this, Increment should be 100mg/day every 1-2 weeks added to the earlier daily dose

Add on to Non enzyme inducing & non Valproic acid

Week 1 & 2: 25mg alternate day

Week 3 & 4: 50mg everyday

Maintenance dose: 225-375/day in 2 divided doses. To achieve this, Increment should be 50mg/day every 1-2 weeks added to the earlier daily dose

LANSOPRAZOLE

Oral

<30Kg: 1mg/kg max 15mg once a day half an hour before feed

>30kg: 15-30mg once a day half an hour before feed

LEVETIRACETAM

Status Epilepticus: as second line drug

> Loading: IV20-30mg/kg dose.   After 12 hours; IV/oral 10mg/kg/dose every 12 hourly. Max 3g/day

Neonatal seizure: 2nd line drug: IV/oral 10-30mg/kg/day

Myoclonic epilepsy, Partial seizures, tonic clonic seizure: Oral 20-30mg/kg/dose 2-3 twice a day

LEVOCETIRIZINE

Children 6-11 years-2.5mg once a day

Children >12 years-5mg once a day

LEVOFLOXACIN

Oral/IV

6months-5 years: 10mg/kg/dose every 12 hours

>5years- 10mg/kg/day single dose. max 500mg/day

LEVO SALBUTAMOL

Asthma

MDI with Spacer device: 2-11 years: 1-2 puffs (50µg=1puff) 4-6 hourly

>12 years: 2-3 puffs 4-6 hourly

Nebulization: <4 years: 0.31-1.25mg every 6-8 hourly

5-11 years: 0.31-0.63mg every 6-8 hours

>12 years: 0.63-1.25mg every 6-8 hourly

Acute Severe asthma

MDI with spacer: 5-18 years: 4-8 puffs every 20 minutes for 3 doses, then every 1-4 hours as needed

Nebulization: 0.075mg/kg every 20 minutes for 3 doses, then 0.075-0.15mg /kg 1-4 hourly as needed

>12 years: 1.25-2.5 mg every 20 minutes for 3 doses, then 1.25-5mg 1-4 hourly as needed

Oral: 2-6 years: 1mg every 8 hourly

6-12years: 2mg every 8 hourly

>12 years 2-4mg every 8 hourly

LEVOTHYROXINE

Oral: morning dose on empty stomach

0-3 months: 10-15mcg/kg

3-6months: 8-10mcg/kg or 25-50mcg

6-12months: 6-8mcg/kg or 50-75mcg

1-5years: 5-6mcg/kg or 75-100mcg

6-12 years: 4-5mcg/kg or 100-125mcg

>12 years: 2-3mcg/kg or >150mcg

LINEZOLID

IV/oral

10mg/kg/dose every 12 hours

LORATIDINE

Oral

Children 2-5 years: 5mg once a day

Children >6 years: 10mg once a day

LORAZEPAM

Anxiety or sedation; oral/IV: 0.02-0.9mg/kg/dose

Status Epilepticus: IV;

Neonates: 0.05mg/kg slow IV over 2-5 minutes, may repeat after 10 minutes

Infants & children: 0.05-0.1mg/kg. Max 4mg, slow IV over 2-5 minutes .may repeat after 10 minutes

Adolescents: 0.07mg/kg Max 8mg .slow IV over 2-5 minutes. May repeat after 10 minutes

LOSARTAN

Hypertension> 6 years initial; 0.7mg/kg max 50 mg. once a day

Reduction of proteinuria in CKD:0.4-0.8mg/kg/day

MAGNESIUM

Elemental Magnesium content of Magnesium salts		
MAGNESIUM SALT	ELEMENTAL MAGNESIUM mg/500mg salt	MAGNESIUM mEq/500mg salt
Magnesium chloride	59	4.9
Magnesium gluconate	27	2.4
Magnesium oxide	302	25
Magnesium l-aspartate	49.6	4.1
Magnesium sulphate	49.3	4.1

RDA

Age	RDA mg/day
<6months	40
6-12 months	60
1-3 years	80
4-8 year	130
9-13 years	Male:240 Female:240
14-18 years	Male:410 Female: 360

MAGNESIUM HYDROXIDE

Constipation:

Children <2years-0.5ml/kg/single dose

Children 2-5 years-5-15ml single bedtime dose

Children 6-11 years-15-30ml single bed time dose

Children >12 years-30-60ml single bedtime dose

MAGNESIUM SUPHATE

1g Magnesium sulphate = 98.6 elemental Magnesium = 8.12mEq Magnesium

Hypomagnesaemia

Neonate: IV 25-50mg MgSo4 /kg/dose every 8-12 hours for 2-3 doses infused over 2 hours

Children: IM/IV: 25-50mg MgSo4/kg/dose every 4-6 hours for 3-4 doses.max 2000mg MgSo4

Daily maintenance: 0.25-0.5mEq magnesium/kg/day. Max 8-24mEq magnesium/day

Management of seizure: IM/IV: 20-100mg Magnesium sulphate /kg/dose every 4-6 hours

Bronchodilation: single dose adjunctive therapy: IV 25-75mg/kg

MANNITOL

Cerebral edema: 0.5-1g/kg initially followed by 0.25-0.5g/kg every 4-6 hours

MEBENDAZOLE

Pin worm: single 100mg dose

Whipworm, roundworm, hookworm: 100mg 2times a day for 3 days

MEDIUM CHAIN TRIGLYCERIDES

Oral

Infants: 0.5ml with alternate feeds, increasing volumes by 0.5ml every 2-3days

Ketogenic diet: 40ml with each meal to achieve 50-75% of total calories

MEFENEMIC ACID

Analgesic & anti pyretic > 6years: 6.5mg/kg/dose every 8 hours

MEFLOQUINE

Oral

Treatment of malaria: 15mg/kg/dose (max 750mg) followed 6-12 hours later by a 10mg/kg/dose (Max 5 00mg)

Prophylaxis: 5mg/kg single dose once a week on the same day.max 250mg/dose

Start 1 week prior to travel & continue till 4 weeks after travel

MEROPENEM

Neonates: 20mg/kg/dose 8-12 hourly

Children >3months: 20mg/kg/dose 8 hourly max dose 1g

Meningitis: 40mg/kg/dose 8hourly max dose 2 g

MESALAMINE

Oral

50mg/kg/day divided every 8-12 hours

METHOTREXATE

JRA: oral: 5-15mg/m2/week or 0.3mg/kg/dose once weekly

Dermatomyositis: oral: 15-20mg/m2/week or 0.3-1mg/kg/dose once weekly

METHYL DOPA

Oral

Initial 10mg/kg/day in 2-4 divided doses max 3g/day

METHYLENE BLUE

Methemoglobinemia: IV 1-2mg/kg may be repeated after 1 hour

Chronic Methemoglobinemia: oral 100mg/day

METHYLPREDNISOLONE

Acute asthma:

Children <12 years

Life threatening emergency medical care: IV 1-2mg/kg/day in 2 divided doses.max 60mg/day

Short course: Oral; 1-2mg/kg/day in 1-2 divided doses. Max 5 days

Children >12 years

Life threatening emergency medical care: IV 40-80 mg/day in 1-2 divided doses

Short course: Oral; 40-60mg/day in1-2 divided doses. Max 5 days

Anti inflammatory or immunosuppressive: oral/IV: 0.5-1.7mg/kg/day in 2-3divided doses

Lupus nephritis: IV: 30mgkg alternate days for 6 doses

Acute spinal cord injury: 30mg/kg over 15minutes, followed in 1hour by a continuous infusion of 5.4mg/kg/hour over 23 hrs.

METOCLOPROMIDE

Anti emetic: Oral/IV: <6years:0.1mg/kg 6-12 years: 2.5-5mg. IV should be infused over 15 minutes

METOPROLOL

Oral: Hypertension: 1-2 mg/kg/day in 2 divided doses

METRONIDAZOLE

Oral/IV/Vaginal cream

Neonates: LBW<2kg: 7.5mg/kg/day once every 24 hours & >2kg every 12 hours

Infants & children: 35-50mg/kg/day in 3 divided doses

H.Pylori: 15-20mg/kg/day in 2 divided doses in combination with2 other agents

Anaerobic infections: IV/oral: 30mg/kg/day in 3 divided doses

MIDAZOLAM

Neonates

Sedation during mechanical ventilation: <32 weeks: 0.03mg/kg/hour

> 32 weeks:0.06mg/kg/hour

Infants >2months-children

Status Epilepticus

 Loading dose: 0.15mg/kg over 2-5minutes followed by a continuous infusion of 1mcg/kg/minute .max 18mcg/kg/min

Sedation: Oral single dose0.25-0.5mg/kg max 20mg

   IV:0.05-0.1mg/kg max6mg

Intra nasal: 0.2mg/kg may repeat after 5-15 minutes

Sedation during mechanical ventilation: Loading dose: 0.05-0.2mg/kg followed by continuous infusion 0.06-0.12mg/kg/hour

MINOCYCLINE

Oral

Children> 8 years: 4mg/kg followed by 2mg/kg/dose every 12 hourly

Children >12years: Acne: 45-59 kg: 45mg once a day; 60-90kg: 90mg once a day

MONTELUKAST

Children 6months- 5 years: 4mg/day

   6-14years: 5mg/day

   >14 years: 10mg/day

NAPROXEN

Oral

Children >2 years

Analgesia: 5-7mg/kg/dose every 8-12 hours

Inflammatory disease: 10-15mg/kg/day in 2 divided doses

NIACIN

AGE	RDA mg/day
<6months	5mg
6months-1 year	6mg
1-3 years	9mg
4-6 years	12mg
7-10years	13mg
Females 11-24 years	15mg/day
Male 11-14 years	17mg/day
Male 15-18 years	20mg/day

Pellagra: 50-100mg/dose 3 times a day

Hyperlipidemia: 100-250mg/day in 3 divided doses

NIFEDIPINE

Hypertensive emergency: oral/sublingual: 0.25-0.5mg/kg/dose.max10mg/dose

NITAZOXANIDE

Oral

Amoebiasis, Giardiasis, Cryptosporidiosis, Helminthiasis:

Children 12-47months:100mg every 12 hours for 3 days

Children 4-11 years: 200mg every 12 hours for 3 days

Children >12 years: 500mg every 12 hours for 3 days

NITILMYCIN

IV

Neonate <1 week: 3mg/kg dose every 12 hourly   >1 week: 3mg/kg dose every 8 hourly

Children: 7.5mg/kg/day in 3 divided doses or single dose.

NITRAZEPAM

Oral

Infantile spasms, Myoclonic epilepsy: initial: 0.25mg/kg in 2 divided doses.

Maintenance 0.5mg/kg/day in 2 divided dosesmax1mg/kg/day.

NITROFURANTOIN

Uncomplicated UTI >3months-12 years: 5-7mg/kg/day

12-18 years: 200-400mg/day in 4 divided doses

UTI prophylaxis: 1-2.5mg/kg one bed time dose.max 100mg/day

NOREPINEPHRINE (NORADRENALINE)

Stimulates α adrenergic receptors (vasoconstrictive) more than β1 adrenergic receptors (Inotropic & chronotropic).

Initial 0.05-0.1mcg/kg/minute. Max 1-2mcg/kg/minute

Central line(mg/kg to be added in 50ml D5)	Peripheral line(mg/kg to be added in 100ml D5) short term use only
0.3mg/kg , 1ml/hr= 0.1µg/kg/minute	0.6mg/kg 1ml/hr= 1µg/kg/min

OCTREOTIDE

Bleeding Varices: 1mcg/kg bolus followed by infusion at 1mcg/kg/hour till bleeding stops.

OFLOXACIN

Oral/IV

10-15mg/kg/day in 2 divided doses

OMEPRAZOLE

Oral

1mg/kg/day once a day 1 hour before food

ONDANSETRON

Oral given half an hour before food

  Children 4-11 years: 1mg three times a day

  Children >11years: 8mg three times a day

IV/IM: 6moths to 18 years:0.1mg/kg/dose

ORAL REHYDRATION SALT (WHO-ORS)

SALT NAME	SALT CONTENT IN 4.4g/Sachet	ELECTROLYTES mOsm/L
Nacl	0.52g	Na 75
KCl	0.30 g	K 20
Na citrate	0.58g	Cl 65
Dextrose anhydrous	2.70g	Citrate 10 Dextrose 75 Total Osmolarity 245

WHO guidelines for ORS in children with no dehydration	
Age	**Quantity to be offered after each stool**
<6months	50ml (quarter cup)
7months-2years	50-100ml (quarter to half cup)
2-5 years	100-200ml (half to one cup)
>5 years	200ml or more (as much as the child can take)

WHO guidelines for ORS in children with some dehydration			
Age	**Wt in kg**	**ORS/day**	**Cup/day**
<4months	<5kg	200-400ml	1-2 cups
4-11 months	5 7.9kg	400 600ml	2-3 cups
12-23months	8-10.9	600-800ml	3-4cups
2-4 years	10-15.9	800-1200ml	4-6cups
5-14 years	16-29.9	1200-2200ml	6-11cups
>15 years	>30kg	>2200ml	12-20cups

OSELTAMIVIR

Treatment of Influenza: should begin within 48hours of onset of symptoms. If initiated after 48 hours it reduces duration of illness & mortality.

<3months:12mg twice a day for 5 days

3-5months:20mg twice a day for 5 days

6-11months:25mg twice a day for 5days

1-12 years: 2mg/kg/dose twice a day max 30mg/dose for 5 days

>12 years: 75mg twice a day for 5 days.

Prophylaxis of influenza: within 2 days of contact to 10 days post contact

< 3months only if critically ill contact

3-5months: 20mg once a day

6-11 months: 25mg once a day

1-12 years: Once a day dose   <15kg: 30mg, 15-23kg: 45mg, 23-40kg: 60mg, >40kg: 75mg

>13years: 75mg once a day

OXCARBAZEPINE

Children 2-16 years

Adjunctive therapy

2-4 years: initial dose 8-10mg/kg/day in 2 divided doses (max 600mg/day) increase to max over 2 weeks 60mg/kg/day

4-16 years: : initial dose 8-10mg/kg/day in 2 divided doses (max 600mg/day) increase over 2 weeks to

Weight dependent dose 20-29kg: 900mg/day in 2 divided doses

30-39kg: 1200mg/day in 2 divided doses

>40kg: 1800mg/day in 2 divided doses

PANTOPRAZOLE

Oral/IV

1mg/kg/day single dose half an hour before feeds

PENICILLAMINE

Oral

Wilson's disease; maintain urinary copper >2mg/kg & free serum copper <10mcg/dl

20mg/kg/day in 2-4 divided doses max 1gm/day

Rheumatoid arthritis; Initial: 3mg/kg/day for 3 months then 6mg/kg/day for 3 months. Given in 3 divided doses

Cystinuria: 30mg/kg/day in 4 divided doses max 4g/day

Lead poisoning

Mild poisoning: 15mg/kg/day   Moderate to severe poisoning: 20-30mg/kg/day

Start with 25% of the dose & increase to the full dose in 2-3 weeks

Arsenic poisoning: 100mg/kg/day divided in 4 daily doses for 5 days. Max 1g/day

PENICILLIN AQUEOUS/PARENTERAL

IV

Neonate: <7 day

<2kg: 50,000u/kg/day every 12 hour divided dose

> 2kg: 75,000/kg/day every 8 hour divided dose

Neonate >7days

1.2-2 kg: 75,000/kg/day every 8 hour divided dose

>2 kg: 100,000u/kg/day every 6 hour divided dose

Congenital syphilis: 150,000u/kg/day in divided doses 8 hourly

Infants & children

100,000u-250,000/kg/day in divided doses 4-6 hourly

Severe infection: 250,000-400,000u/kg/day in divided doses 4-6 hourly max 24million u/day

PENICILLIN BENZATHINE

Deep IM

Neonates: congenital syphilis: 50,000u/kg single dose

Infants & children:

Group A Streptococcal upper respiratory tract infection: 25,000-50,000/kg as single dose.

Max 1.2 million units/dose

Prophylaxis against Rheumatic Fever: 50,000u/kg single dose every 21 days max 1.2 million units /dose

Syphilis: 50,000u/kg every week for 3 weeks. Max 2.4 million units/dose

PERMETHRIN

Topical

Head lice: 1% crème: wash hair with shampoo & dry. Apply Permethrin crème to hair. Wash off after 10minutes. Fine comb to remove nits. May repeat after 1 week

Scabies: infants: apply 5% cream at bed time all over the body. Leave6 hours &wash off.

Children: apply 5% cream at bed time all over the body. Leave 12 hours &wash off

PHENOBARBITONE

Anticonvulsant:

Status Epilepticus: Loading dose

Neonates: 15-20mg/kg/dose may repeat after 15-20minutes. Max 40mg/kg/day

Infants & children: 15-20mg/kg/dose (max1000mg dose) may repeat after 15-20minutes.

Max 40mg/kg/day

Maintenance dose

Oral/IV

To start 12 hours after the loading dose

Neonates: 3-5mg/kg/day single dose

Infants: 5mg/kg/day in 2 divided doses

Children: 1-5 years: 6-8mg/kg/day 1-2 divided doses

Children 5-12 years: 4-6mg/kg/day1-2 divided doses

Children >12 years: 1-3mg/kg/day 1-2 divided doses

Sedation: Children: Oral 2mg/kg 3times a day

Hyperbilirubinemia: Oral: 3-8mg/kg/day in2-3 divided doses

PHENYLEPHRINE

Oral: nasal decongestant

2-5 years: 2.5ml every 8 hourly

>5 years: 5ml every 8 hourly

PHENYTOIN

Status Epilepticus; IV

Neonates, Infants& children: 15-20mg/kg/dose

 20ml/kg dissolve in 20ml NS & infuse over 20-30minutes.May repeat after 30 minutes

Maintenance: IV/oral: start after12 hours of loading dose

 Neonates, Infants & Children 5mg/kg/day in 2-3 divided doses

PIPERACILLIN TAZOBACTAM

IV dose based on mg of Piperacillin.max 16g of Piperacillin

Infants<6months:150-300mg/kg/day in divided 6-8 hourly doses

Infants >6months & children: 240mg/kg/day in 8 hourly divided doses

Severe pseudomonas infection: 300-400mg/kg/day in 6 hourly divided doses

Appendicitis /Peritonitis: 240-300mg/kg/day in 8 hourly divided doses

POLYETHYLENE GLYCOL 3350

Oral

Constipation > 4 years: 0.7-1.5g/kg daily single dose max 17g/day added to 125-250ml of water or juice.

POTASSIUM BICARBONATE & POTASSIUM CHLORIDE/CITRATE

Oral

Prevention of hypokalemia & treatment (serum K is >3.5mEq/l)1-2mEqkg/day in 2 divided doses. 20ml=15mEq Potassium

POTASSIUM CHLORIDE

IV

Hypokalemia

Serum K is <3mEq/l: increase the potassium in the IVfluids

Serum K is <2.5mEq/L:

Neonates, infants & children:

Intermittent infusion: diluted:0.5-1mEq/kg/dose (max40mEq) at 0.3-0.5mEq/kg/hour max1mEq/kg/hour

PREDNISOLONE

Oral

Asthma

Children<12years

Acute exacerbations: 1-2mg/kg/day in 2 divided doses (max 60mg/day)

Short course: 1-2mg/kg/day in 2 divided doses for 3-10 days

Long course: 0.25-2mg/kg/ single daily dose

Children > 12 years

Acute exacerbations: 40-80mg /day in 1-2 divided doses

Short course: 40-60mg/day in 1-2 divided doses for 3-10 days

Long course: 7.5-60mg/day single daily dose

Anti inflammatory/immunosuppressive: 0.1-2mg.kg/day in 1-4 divided doses

Nephrotic syndrome:

Induction: 2mg/kg/day in 1-3 divided doses.max 80mg/day for 6 weeks, followed by 2mg/kg/alternate day single morning dose for 6 weeks

Relapse: 2mg/kg/day in 1-3 divided doses for 2 weeks followed by 2mg/kg/single dose alternate days for 6weeks

Frequent relapses: 0.5-1mg/kg/dose alternate days for 3-6 months

PRIMAQUIN

Oral: Given once a day for 14 days, start from the day 4 of anti malarial therapy

1-12 years: 0.25mg/kg

>12 years: 15mg.

PROMETHAZINE

Children>2years

Antihistamine: oral:0.1mg/kg/dose (max12.5mg) every 6hours

Antiemetic: oral: oral/IM 0.25-1mg/kg max 25mg. 4 times a day

Motion sickness: oral: 0.5mg/kg max 50mg, 30-60minutes prior to departure.

Sedation: oral/IM:0.5-1mg/kg/dose max 50mg, every 6 hours

PROPRANOLOL

Neonates: oral:0.25mg/kg/dose every 6-8 hours

IV: 0.01mg/kg slow infusion over 10minutes may be repeated after 6-8 hours

Arrhythmias: Oral:0.5-4mg/kg/day in divided doses 6-8 hourly

IV:0.01-0.1mg/kg slow IV over 10 minutes. Max; infants: 1mg, children:3mg

Hypertension: oral: initial dose-0.5-1mg/kg/day in 2-4 divided doses, increase to 1-5mg/kg/day in 2-4 divided doses if needed

Migraine prophylaxis: 1mg/kg/day divided every 8 hourly

Cyanotic spell (Tetrology of Fallot): Oral: begin with 0.25mg/kg/dose every 6 hourly,

if needed can be increased to maximum 5mg/kg/day

IV: 0.01-0.02mg/kg/dose infused over 10 minutes

Thyrotoxicosis: Neonates & children: oral: 2mg/kg/day in divided doses every 6-12 hours

Adolescents: 10-40mg/dose every 6 hours

PSEUDOEPHIDRINE

Children< 2years: Oral: 4mg/kg/day in divided doses 6 hourly

2-5years: oral: 15mg every 6 hourly

6-12 years: oral: 30mg every 6 hourly

>12 years: oral: 60mg every 6 hourly

PYRAZINAMIDE: Oral:15-40mg/kg/day single dose max 2g/day

PYRIDOSTIGMINE

Myasthenia gravis: oral: Neonates: 5mg every 4-6 hours

Children: 7mg/kg/day in 6 divided doses

PYRIDOXINE

AGE	RDA
<6months	0.1mg
6-12 months	0.3mg
1-3 years	0.5mg
4-8 years	0.6mg
9-13 years	1mg
14-19 years	1.3mg

Pyridoxine dependent seizures: Oral/IM/IV: 10-100mg/day

Dietary deficiency: oral: 5-25mg/day for 3 Weeks, then 1.5-2.5mg/day

Drug induced neuritis: Oral: Treatment: 10-50mg/day   Prophylaxis: 1-2mg/kg/day

Isoniazid poisoning: Total dose equivalent to the amount of Isoniazid ingested. 1-4gm IV followed by 1gm IM every 30 minutes to complete the dose

Mushroom poisoning: IV 25mg/kg .Repeat if needed.

QUININE

Chloroquine resistant malaria: Oral: 30mg/kg/day divided doses 8 hourly for7 days in conjunction with other agents.max 2g/day

Babesiosis: 25mg/kg/day divided every 8 hourly for 7-10 days .max 650mg/dose

RANITIDINE

Oral/IV/IV infusion

Infants<1month: oral: 2mg/kg/day in divided doses every 12 hours

IV:1.5-2mg/kg/day in divided doses every 12 hours

Children> 1 month to 16 years: oral: 4-8mg/kg/day in divided doses every 12 hours

Max 300mg/day

IV:1.5mg/kg/dose every 12 hourly

RIBAVIRIN

Chronic hepatitis C in combination with interferon 2bα: 15mg/kg/day in 2 divided doses

SACCHROMYCES BOULARDII

250mg/5 billion spores 2-3 times a day

SALMETEROL

Children >4 years

Maintenance & prevention of asthma: inhalation: 1 puff (50mcg) every 12 hours in conjunction with inhaled steroids

Prevention of exercise induced asthma: 1 puff (50mcg) 30minutes before exercise.

SILDENAFIL

Pulmonary Hypertension

IV:

Neonates:0.5-1mg/kg/dose every 6 hours

Infants & children: 0.25-2 mg/kg dose every 4 hours

SIMETHICONE

Infants & children < 2years: 20mg/4 times a day

Children 2-12 years: 40mg/4 times a day

Children > 12 years: 40-250mg after meals 4 times a day

SODIUM BENZOATE

Adjunctive treatment of treatment of hyper ammonemia: Oral/IV

Infants & children: 0.25mg/kg bolus followed by 0.25g/kg/day as divided doses every 6-8 hours

SODIUM BICARBONATE

Cardiac arrest: child should be on ventilation before administering $NaHCO_3$

Infants & children: 1mEq/kg in 10 minutes. If needed next dose after 10 minutes 0.5mEq/kg based on acid base balance

Metabolic acidosis

To be used administered only after other standard treatment measures have been used

If acid bade status is not available: older children: 2-5mEq/kg infused over 4-8 hours

Based on acid base balance: $HCO_3 mEq = 0.3 \times wt$ in kg $\times$ base deficit mEq

Correction to done over 2 hours

Prevention hyperuricemia secondary to Tumor lysis syndrome (urinary alkalinization):

IV: 120-200mEq/m2/day diluted in 3000ml of maintenance fluids to keep urinary pH 6-7

Oral: 12g/m2/day in 4 divided doses to keep urinary pH 6-7

Renal Tubular Acidosis

Distal: 2-3mEq/kg/day (84-840mg/day) in 4 divided doses

Proximal: 5-10mEq/kg/day in 4 divided doses

Injection solution	Bicarbonate content
4.2%	5mEq/10ml
7.5%	8.9mEq/10ml
8.4%	10mEq/10ml

SODIUM CHLORIDE

Maintenance sodium requirements:

Premature neonates: 2-8mEq/kg/day

Term neonates: 1-4mEq/kg/day

Infants & children: 3-4mEq/kg/day max 100-150mEq/day

Correction of Asymptomatic Hyponatremia: do not exceed a correction rate of 8-10mEq/L per day

Correction of symptomatic Hyponatremia (seizures, coma): Infusion of 3% Nacl at a dose of

2-3ml/kg over 1Hour

mEq sodium = (desired sodium 125mEq/L- actual sodium mEq/L) × 0.6 ×weight in kg

Solution	Na mEq/l	Cl mEq/l	Osmolaririty	Tonicity
¼ NS (0.25%) +D5	34	34	329	Hypotonic
½ NS (0.5%)	77	77	154	Hypotonic
NS	154	154	308	Isotonic
3% NS	513	513	1026	Hypertonic

SPIRONOLACTONE

Oral

Neonate: Diuretic: 1-3mg/kg/day in 1-2 divided doses

Children: Diuretic, Hypertension: 1-3.3mg/kg/day in 6-12 hour divided doses max 100mg/day

Monitor serum K levels on Day 3, 8 & then every 2-3 months. Stop therapy if serum K>5mEq/l or serum creatinine > 4mg/dl

STREPTOMYCIN

IM

Neonates: 10-20mg/kg/once a day

Infants: 20-30mg/kg/day in2 divided doses

Tuberculosis: 20-40mg/kg/once a day for 1 month. Max 1g/day. Monitor for tinnitus & impaired hearing.

SUCRALFATE

Oral

40-80mg/kg/day in divided doses 6 hourly. Should be taken 1 hour before meals.

SULFAMETHOXAZOLE & TRIMETHOPRIM

Dose as per Trimethoprim content

Children> 2months:

Mild – moderate infections: 6-12 mg TMP /kg/day in 2 divided doses

Serious infection /Pneumocystis: 15-20mg/kg/day in divided doses 6-8 hours

Prophylaxis of Pneumocystis: 150mg/m2/day in 2 divided doses, on 3 consecutive days of the week

 Max: 320mg TMX

Prevention of UTI: 2mg TMP/kg/day as single dose

SULFASALAZINE

Oral

Children >2 years: Ulcerative colitis

Mild exacerbation: 40-50mg/kg/day in divided 6 hourly doses

Moderate to severe exacerbation: 50-75mg/kg/day in divided 6 hourly doses Max 6g/day

Maintenance dose: 30-50mg/kg/day max 2g/day

JRA: start therapy with 10mg/kg/day in 2 divided doses. Increase weekly to reach

30-50mg/kg/day in 2 divided doses max dose 2g/day

SUMATRIPTAN

Oral/Intranasal

Acute Migraine

6-10 years: 25mg   10-12 years: 50mg   12-18 years: 50-100mg as single dose.

Dose may be repeated after 1 hour.

TACROLIMUS

IV/ Oral: to be given in a glass cup only

Transplant	Route of dose	Initial dose of Tacrolimus
Liver	Oral	0.15-0.2mg/kg/day in 2 doses
	IV	0.03-0.05mg/kg/day as infusion
Kidney	Oral	0.2-0.3mg/kg/day in 2 doses
	IV	0.06mg/kg/day as infusion

Topical in Moderate to severe atopic dermatitis: 0.03% cream. Apply twice a day

TEICOPLANIN

IV infusion over 30 minutes

Neonate: Initial: 16mg/kg, after 24 hours start maintenance dose of 8mg/kg/day as single dose

Children: 10mg/kg/dose 2 times a day for 3 doses, then once daily

TERBINAFINE

Tinea capitis & Onychomycosis: Oral: 125-250mg/day single dose for 6 weeks

Topical: apply twice a week for 1week

TERBUTALINE

Children<12 years

  Oral: 0.05-0.15mg/kg/dose every 8 hours max 5mg/day

   SubQ: 0.005-0.01mg/kg/dose max0.4mg/dose. Can be repeated every 20minutes for 3 doses only. Can be repeated after 4 hours

Children>12 years

  Oral: 2.5-5mg/kg/dose ever 8 hours.max 7.5-10mg/day

  SubQ: 0.25mg/dose. Can be repeated after 20 minutes for 3 doses only.

TESTOSTERONE

Deep IM .max dose 400mg

Male Hypogonadism

Initiation of pubertal growth: 40-50mg/m2/dose monthly, until the growth rate fall to pre pubertal level

Terminal growth phase: 100mg/m2/dose monthly, until the growth ceases

Maintenance virilizing dose: 100mg/m2 twice monthly

Delayed puberty: 40-50mg/m2/dose monthly for 6 months

TETRACYCLINE

Children > 8 Years: oral: 25-50mg /kg/day in 4 divided doses. Max 3g/day

For Rickettsia, Brucella, Chlamydia, Acne vulgaris, Lyme disease, Legionella

THEOPHYLLINE

Oral: 6weeks – 6months: 10mg/kg/day in 3 divided doses

      6months to 1 Year: 12-18mg/kg/day in 3 divided doses

      Children 1-9 years: 20-24mg/kg in 3 divided doses

      Children 9-12 years: 16mg/kg/day in 3 divided doses

      Children 12-16 years: 13mg/kg/day in 3 divided doses

THIAMINE

AGE	RDA mg/day
1-3 years	0.5
4-8 years	0.6
9-13	0.9
14-18	1-1.2mg

Thiamine deficiency

Critically ill (Wernicke's encephalopathy, cardiac effects): IV / IM10-25mg/dose 3 times a day

Otherwise oral: 10-50mg/dose daily for 2 weeks then 5-10mg/day for 1 month

TOBRAMYCIN

IM/IV

Preterm /wt <1200gm: 2.5mg/kg/dose every 18 hours

1200-2000gm: 2.5mg/kg/dose every 12 hours

>2000gm:2.5mg/kg/dose every 8 hours

Infants &Children < 5years:2.5mg/kg/dose every 8 hours

Children > 5years: 2.5mg/kg/dose every 8hours

TOPIRAMATE

Adjunctive anticonvulsant therapy: Oral

Children 2-16 years

Partial onset seizures or Lennox-Gastaut syndrome: initial: 1-3mg/kg/day as night dose max 25mg. Increase dose at 1-2 week intervals by 1-3mg/kg/day to 5-9mg/kg/day in 2 divided doses.

Primary Generalized tonic clonic seizures: initial: 1-3mg/kg/day as night dose max 25mg. Increase slowly to reach 6mg/kg/day in 2 divided doses by 8 weeks.

TOPICAL STEROIDS

CLASSIFICATION & POTENCY	NAME OF STEROID
Class 1 Very high potency	0.05% Clobetasol propionate cream/ointment 0.05% Halobetasol propionate cream/ointment 0.05% Betamethasone dipropionate cream/ointment
Class 2 High potency	0.25% Desoximetasone cream/ointment 0.1% Mometasone furoate ointment
Class 3 Medium potency	0.05% Betamethasone dipropionate cream 0.05% Fluocinonide cream 0.05% Desoximetasone cream 0.1% Betamethasone valerate ointment 0.005% Fluticasone ointment
Class4 Medium Potency	0.1% Mometasone furoate cream 0.1% Triamcinolone acetonide cream/ointment 0.1% Betamethasone valerate cream 0.025% Fluocinolone acetonide ointment
Class 5 Lower medium potency	0.05% Fluticasone propionate cream/lotion 0.1% Triamcinolone acetonide cream/lotion 0.025% Fluocinolone cream 0.1% Hydrocortisone butyrate cream/ointment
Class 6 Low potency	0.05% Desonide cream 0.1% Hydrocortisone butyrate lotion 0.025% Triamcinolone acetonide lotion 0.01% Fluocinolone acetonide lotion 0.1% Betamethasone valerate lotion
Class 7 Lowest potency	Hydrocortisone acetate Cream

TRAMADOL

Oral/IM

1-2mg/kg/dose every 6 hourly .max 400mg/day

Adolescents: 50-100mg every 6 hourly max 400mg/day

TRANEXAMIC ACID

In Hemophilia in conjunction with replacement therapy

IV: 10mg/kg immediately before surgery & then 1omg/kg/dose every 6-8 hours for 2-8 days

URSODIOL (Ursodeoxycholic acid)

Biliary Artesia cholestasis: 10mg/kg/once a day

Hepatitis cholestasis: 30mg/kg/day in 2 divided doses

TPN cholestasis: 30mg/kg/day in 3 divided doses

Gall stones: 5mg/kg/single dose for 6months to 1year

VALPROIC ACID

Seizure disorder: initial: oral 10-15mg/kg/day in 1-3 divided dose. Increase if needed at weekly intervals to reach maintenance dose of 30-60mg/kg/day

Refractory Status Epilepticus: IV 20-40mg/kg dilute in 50ml NS & infuse over 1 hour

IV maintenance dose is the equivalent to oral maintenance dose

Rectal: Dilute syrup1:1 with water & use as retention enema: initial: 17-20mg/kg, maintenance 10-15mg/kg/dose every 8 hours

VANCOMYCIN

IV

Neonates

<7 days ;< 1.2kg: 15mg/kg/day every 24 hours

     1.2-2kg: 15mg/kg/day every 12-18 hours

     >2 kg: 15mg/kg/day every 12 hours

> 7 days: 15-20mg/kg/day every 8 hours

Infants >1month & children: 40mg/kg/day in 6-8 hourly divided doses

Staphylococcus Meningitis/CNS infection: 60mg/kg/day in divided 6 hourly doses

Max .1g/dose

IV intermittent infusion over 60minutes should be used. Rapid infusion produces Red Man Syndrome (red rash over head & upper trunk, intense pruritus, tachycardia, hypotension)

If a maculopapular rash develops slow the rate of infusion to 90-120 minutes.

Administration of anti-histaminic prior to infusion reduces /prevents the reaction

VITAMIN E

Age	RDA mg/day
0-6 months	4units
7-12 months	6 units
1-3 years	6units
4-8 years	7units
9-13 years	11units
>14 years	15 units

1 unit Vitamin E= 1mg α tocopherol acetate

Oral

Vitamin E deficiency

Neonates: 25-50 units /day

Children: 1unit/kg/day

Prevention of Vitamin E deficiency: Neonates: 5mg/day

WARFARIN

Oral/IV

To maintain an INR between 2-3

Initial: 0.2mg/kg

Maintenance dose: 0.1mg/kg/day as single daily dose

IV: 5mg dilute with 2.7ml water for injection, slow injection over 1-2 minutes into peripheral vein

ZINC SUPPLEMENTS

AGE	ELEMENTAL ZINC mg/day
<12 months	5mg
1-10 years	10mg
>11 years	12-15mg

Zinc deficiency:

0.5-1mg elemental zinc /day in 1-3 divided doses

Clinical response may occur after 6-8 weeks of treatment.

Diarrhea

< 6months: 10mg elemental zinc for 14 days

>6months: 20mg elemental zinc

DRUGS THAT CAN CAUSE ERYTHEMA MULTIFORME	
ANTIBIOTICS	Sulphonamides, Tetracycline, Ampicillin, Amoxycillin
NSAIDs	Ibuprofen
ANTICONVULSANTS	Phenytoin, Phenobarbitone

DRUGS TO AVOID IN G6PD DEFICIENCY – DEFINITE RISK OF HEMOLYSIS	
Anti Helminthic	Niridazole
Antibiotics	Sulphonamides Nitrofurantoin, Nitrofurazone Quinolones Chloramphenicol Furazolidone
Anti Malarial	Primaquin
Anti Methhemoglobinimic agent	Methylene blue
Anti Mycobacterials	Dapsone Para amino salicylic acid Isoniazid
Anti Neoplastic drugs	Doxorubicin
Genitourinary analgesic	Pyridium
Anti Convulsants	Phenytoin
Others	Phenyl hydrazine Fava beans, Naphthalene

BREAST FEEDING TO BE AVOIDED WITH INTAKE OF THE FOLLOWING DRUGS BY THE MOTHER	
Cytotoxic drugs	Cyclophosphamide, Cyclosporine,Doxorubicin,Methotrexate
Drugs of abuse	Amphetamines,Cocaine,Heroin,Marijuana,Phenyciclidine
Psychotropic drugs	*Antianxiety*: Alprazolam,Diazepam,Lorazepam,Midazolam *Antidepressant*:Amitrytaline,Amoxapine,Bupropion,Clomipramine,Desipramine,Doxepin Fluoxtine,Imipramine,Nortryptiline,Paroxitine,Sertraline,Trazodone *Antipsychotic*:Chlorpromazine,Clozapine,Haloperidol,Mesoridazine,Trifluoperazine
Radioactive compounds	Copper 64, Gallium 67,Indium111, Iodine;123,125,131, Technetium 99m
Other drugs	Amiodrone,Chloramphenicol,Clofazimine,Lamotrigine,Metoclopromide,Metronidazole, Tinidazole,Lithium,Phenobarbitone,Ergotamine,Clemastine

.

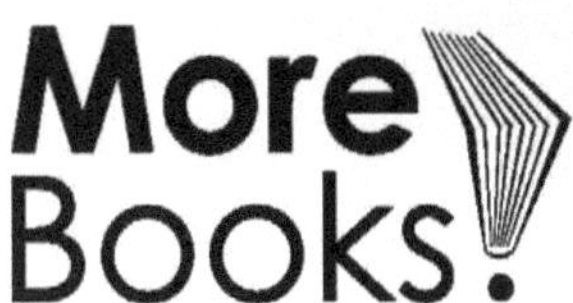

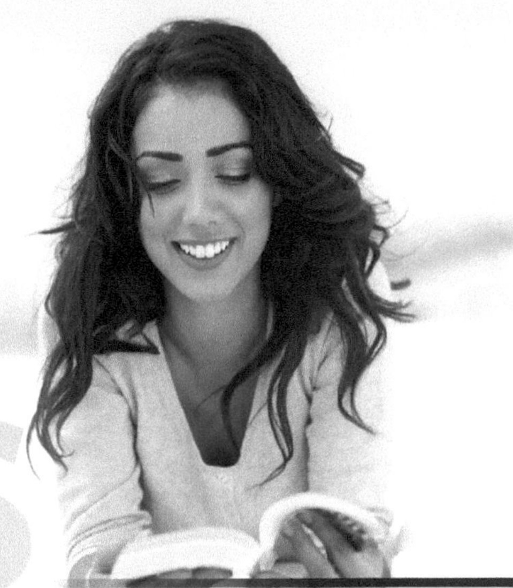

Buy your books fast and straightforward online - at one of the world's fastest growing online book stores! Environmentally sound due to Print-on-Demand technologies.

Buy your books online at

www.get-morebooks.com

Kaufen Sie Ihre Bücher schnell und unkompliziert online – auf einer der am schnellsten wachsenden Buchhandelsplattformen weltweit!
Dank Print-On-Demand umwelt- und ressourcenschonend produziert.

Bücher schneller online kaufen

www.morebooks.de

Printed by Books on Demand GmbH, Norderstedt / Germany